BREASTFEEDING

BENEFITS, CHALLENGES, TIPS, AND SUPPORT

DR. J.P JUDE

Table of Contents

CHAPTER ONE

INTRODUCTION

The natural process of providing an infant with milk from the mother's breasts is called breastfeeding, or nursing. In the early stages of life, breast milk supplies vital nutrients, antibodies, and immune factors that support the baby's growth, development, health, and well-being. Breastfeeding has several advantages for both the mother and the child. It builds a special relationship, connection, and loving experience that supports the baby's emotional, physical, psychological, and developmental needs as well as the mother's.

Overview of breastfeeding:

Composition of Breast Milk:

Nutritional Value: Depending on the baby's growth stage, nutritional demands, and feeding requirements, breast milk provides proteins, lipids, carbs, vitamins, minerals, and antibodies—all of which are necessary for the baby's optimum growth, development, and health.

immunological factors: Antibodies, immunological factors, enzymes, and protective compounds found in breast milk help a baby's immune system fight off infections and illnesses while also boosting general health, resiliency, and wellbeing.

Optimal nourishment: A baby's physical and mental development, as well as their growth and development, are all supported by breastfeeding, which provides full, balanced nourishment.

Immune Support: Breast milk strengthens an infant's defenses against infections, illnesses, allergies, and diseases. It also promotes general health, forbearance, and immunity.

Digestive Health: Breastfeeding lowers discomfort and discomfort associated with digestion while promoting optimal food absorption, metabolism, and gut health.

Bonding and Comfort: Breastfeeding improves the nurturing, love, responsiveness, and maternal-infant relationship between the mother and her child by fostering bonding, connection, attachment, comfort, security, warmth, and emotional well-being.

Advantages of breastfeeding for mothers

Postpartum Recovery: Breastfeeding encourages uterine contraction, lessens bleeding, aids in weight loss, and restores hormonal balance following childbirth. It also promotes healing and recuperation following childbirth.

Benefits to Health: Breastfeeding supports the health, well-being, and lifespan of mothers by lowering the risk of postpartum depression, ovarian cancer, breast cancer, osteoporosis, cardiovascular illnesses, and chronic disorders.

Bonding and Emotional Well-being: Breastfeeding increases maternal bonding, connection, love, responsiveness, confidence, self-esteem, empowerment, and psychological well-being, supporting positive maternal-infant contact, attachment, and relationship.

Breastfeeding Considerations and Practices:

Breastfeeding Techniques: To promote efficient, comfortable, and successful breastfeeding experiences, milk transfer, and feeding sessions, learn and put into practice various breastfeeding positions, latches, holds, feeding signals, rhythms, patterns, and practices.

Breastfeeding Challenges: Providing support, education, interventions, and lactation consultation to promote breastfeeding success, confidence, and well-being while addressing and managing breastfeeding challenges, concerns, issues, difficulties, discomfort, pain, latch problems, engorgement, mastitis, low milk supply, over supply, tongue tie, lip tie, nursing strikes, teething, and transitions.

Breastfeeding Support: Seeking and obtaining from healthcare providers, lactation specialists, counselors, educators, and breastfeeding advocates breastfeeding support, education, resources, guidance, counseling, lactation consultation, community, peer support, groups, and assistance in order to nurture breastfeeding knowledge, skills, confidence, resilience, and well-being throughout the breastfeeding journey, challenges, growth, transitions, and life stages.

Breastfeeding is a natural, caring, and beneficial activity that encourages optimal nutrition, health, growth, bonding, connection, and well-being for infants and mothers. Embracing breastfeeding with knowledge, preparation, support, empowerment, resilience, positivity, connection, and holistic well-being facilitates successful, comfortable, and fulfilling breastfeeding experiences, growth, adaptation, challenges, and life transitions, celebrating the unique, transformative, and nurturing journey of breastfeeding, motherhood, infancy, and life's unfolding chapters.

Benefits of Breastfeeding

Breastfeeding offers significant benefits for both newborns and mothers, encouraging optimal health, development, well-being, bonding, and caring experiences throughout the breastfeeding journey and beyond. Understanding the multifaceted advantages of breastfeeding highlights the importance, value, and impact of breastfeeding on individual and collective health, growth, relationships, and life experiences, fostering informed decisions, support, promotion, and celebration of breastfeeding practices, knowledge, and advocacy.

Advantages of Breastfeeding Young Children:

Superiority in Nutrition:

Complete Nutrition: All the nutrients needed for a baby to grow, develop, and be healthy are found in breast milk. It is balanced, optimum, and full of proteins, lipids, carbs, vitamins, minerals, and antibodies.

Adaptive Composition: Throughout infancy, breast milk supports the baby's optimal development, metabolism, and health by adjusting to match their changing nutritional needs, growth stages, and feeding needs.

Support for the Immune System:

Antibodies and Immunity: Immune components, antibodies, enzymes, and protective compounds found in breast milk strengthen an infant's defenses against infections and illnesses while also fostering general health, resiliency, and wellbeing.

Gut Health and Microbiome: Throughout infancy and adulthood, breastfeeding supports immune system function, digestion, absorption, metabolism, and gut health by promoting a balanced, diverse, and healthy microbiome.

Advantages for Development and Cognition:

Brain Development: Through optimum nutrition, growth factors, and nurturing experiences during early life stages, breastfeeding improves healthy brain development, cognitive function, neurodevelopment, learning, memory, and intellectual ability.

Coordination and Fine and Gross Motor abilities: Through engaging feeding experiences, stimulation, and caring relationships, breastfeeding supports the development of fine and gross motor abilities as well as coordination, strength, agility, mobility, and physical development.

Prevention of Illnesses and Health:

Decreased Infections and Illnesses: Breastfeeding supports general health, vitality, and well-being by lowering the risk of infections, respiratory illnesses, gastrointestinal disorders, ear infections, urinary tract infections, allergies, asthma, and other ailments.

Long-Term Health Benefits: Breastfeeding fosters resilience, health, and wellness through all the stages, changes, and challenges of life. It also provides protection against obesity, diabetes, cardiovascular disease, and chronic diseases.

Psychological and Emotional Health:

Bonding and Attachment: Breastfeeding improves the nurturing, love, responsiveness, and maternal-infant relationship between the mother and her child by fostering bonding, connection, attachment, comfort, security, warmth, and emotional well-being.

Emotional Regulation and Comfort: Through caring interactions, physical proximity, warmth, and the mother-infant bond, breastfeeding promotes emotional regulation, soothing, calming, comfort, stress reduction, relaxation, and emotional health.

Mothers' Advantages of Breastfeeding:

Postpartum Recuperation and Menstruation:

Uterine Contraction and Bleeding Reduction: Breastfeeding supports physical healing, recovery, and mother well-being by promoting uterine contraction, bleeding reduction, postpartum recovery, weight loss, and hormonal balance following childbirth.

Hormonal balance and mood enhancement: During the postpartum period and beyond, breastfeeding promotes psychological well-being, oxytocin release, stress reduction, anxiety alleviation, mood enhancement, and prevention of postpartum depression.

Prevention of Illnesses and Health:

Lower Cancer Risks: Breastfeeding promotes mother health, wellbeing, longevity, and illness prevention by lowering the risk of breast cancer, ovarian cancer, uterine cancer, and other malignancies.

Protection against Chronic illnesses: Breastfeeding promotes general health, wellness, and resilience through life's transitions, phases, and challenges while providing protection against osteoporosis, cardiovascular illnesses, metabolic disorders, and chronic conditions.

CHAPTER TWO

Emotional Health and Bonding:

Maternal Bonding and Connection: Positive mother-infant interaction, attachment, and relationship are fostered by breastfeeding, which also improves maternal bonding, connection, love, responsiveness, confidence, self-esteem, empowerment, and psychological well-being.

Nurturing Experiences: Throughout the breastfeeding journey, struggles, growth, changes, and life stages, breastfeeding supports emotional connection, maternal instincts, intuition, and well-being for mothers. It also provides comforting, soothing, relaxing, and bonding experiences.

Throughout the nursing journey, early life stages, and beyond, breastfeeding promotes optimal nutrition, health, development, bonding, and well-being for both mothers and newborns. The successful, fulfilling, and nurturing breastfeeding experiences, growth, adaptation, challenges, and life transitions are fostered by embracing breastfeeding with knowledge, preparation, support, empowerment, resilience, positivity, connection, and holistic well-being. This approach also celebrates the special, transformative, and nurturing journey of breastfeeding, motherhood, infancy, and life's unfolding chapters.

The Lactation Physiology

In order to feed the baby, the mammary glands produce, secrete, and expel milk throughout the complicated physiological process known as lactation. Throughout the nursing experience, a multitude of hormonal, neural, and local elements collaborate to stimulate, control, and sustain milk production, flow, and composition, all of which are integral parts of the lactation physiology. Comprehending the complex mechanics and phases of lactation offers valuable understanding of the dynamic, adaptive, and responsive nature of the nursing breast to the infant's requirements, promoting the best possible breastfeeding experiences, results, and health for both moms and infants.

Physiology of Breastfeeding:

Control of Hormones:

Prolactin: The anterior pituitary gland's hormone prolactin is essential for promoting lactogenesis, or the production of milk, in the mammary glands. When an infant sucks and empties the breasts, high levels of prolactin during pregnancy and the postpartum period start and maintain milk synthesis.

Oxytocin: The posterior pituitary gland secretes oxytocin, which causes the myoepithelial cells that surround the alveoli and ducts to contract. This contraction results in milk ejection, or the release of milk from the nursing breast in response to the stimulation, feeding cues, and nursing infants sucking.

Progesterone and estrogen: High progesterone and estrogen levels during pregnancy aid in the development of the mammary glands, the expansion of the ducts, and the lactation readiness process. Following childbirth, lactogenesis and milk production can begin and progress into mature milk synthesis due to a decrease in these hormones.

Human Placental Lactogen (hPL): The placenta secretes this substance throughout pregnancy, which aids in the growth of the breasts, the formation of colostrum, and the early secretion of milk in preparation for breastfeeding.

Anatomy of the Breast and Milk Production:

Alveoli and Lobules: The milk-producing organs of the mammary glands are groups of alveoli and lobules. During lactation, milk is synthesized, stored, and secreted into the ducts by milk-producing epithelial cells that line tiny sac-like structures called alveoli.

The ductal system is made up of a network of ducts that carry milk from the alveoli to the nipple. This system enables the flow, storage, and delivery of milk to the baby while nursing.

Myoepithelial cells: During feeding and expression, myoepithelial cells surround the alveoli and ducts and contract in response to the release of oxytocin, facilitating the ejection, flow, and expulsion of milk from the breast.

The composition and synthesis of milk:

Production of Colostrum: The mammary glands generate colostrum, a concentrated and nutrient-rich fluid, in the early postpartum phase. Colostrum supports the newborn's initial eating, immunity, and health by supplying it with proteins, vitamins, minerals, and immunological components.

After colostrum, transitional milk develops into mature milk production, composition, and supply. It does this by adjusting to the infant's changing nutritional needs, growth stages, and feeding requirements in the first few weeks of breastfeeding.

Mature Milk: Made comprised of both foremilk and hindmilk, mature milk is created in response to breastfeeding patterns, stimulation, and suckling of the infant. It offers full, balanced, and ideal nourishment to promote a child's healthy growth, development, and well-being during infancy.

Mechanisms of Neurology and Reflexology:

Suckling Reflex: When a newborn is breastfed, milk flow, and infant feeding are all made easier because nursing stimulates nerve endings in the nipple and areola, which in turn sets off brain pathways and reflex mechanisms that signal the release of oxytocin and milk ejection.

Milk Removal, Breast Emptying, and Milk Production Feedback Mechanisms: Based on infant demand, feeding frequency, milk removal, and breastfeeding patterns, these feedback mechanisms adjust milk supply, composition, and flow to maintain optimal milk production, availability, and quality throughout the breastfeeding journey.

The mammary glands' ability to create, control, and supply nutritious milk to support infant growth, development, health, and well-being during the breastfeeding journey is made possible by the amazing and dynamic process known as lactation physiology. In order to facilitate milk synthesis, secretion, ejection, and delivery in response to infant needs, stimulation, and feeding cues, hormonal regulation, breast anatomy, milk production mechanisms, and neurological reflexes work in concert. This promotes successful, adaptive, and responsive breastfeeding experiences, outcomes, and connections between mothers and babies throughout infancy and life's unfolding chapters. The unique, transformative journey of breastfeeding, motherhood, infancy, and life's evolving experiences are nurtured when one embraces the physiology of lactation with knowledge, preparation, support, empowerment, resilience, positivity, connection, and holistic well-being.

Beginning the Breastfeeding Process

Beginning to breastfeed is an exciting and life-changing experience that calls for planning, education, practice, and support to ensure that moms and babies have successful, comfortable, and satisfying nursing experiences. Throughout the breastfeeding journey, obstacles, growth, changes, and the unfolding chapters of life, embracing breastfeeding with confidence, patience, resilience, connection, and holistic well-being fosters caring connections, bonding, interactions, and adaptations.

Starting a Breastfeeding Journey:

Pregnancy Education and Planning:

Breastfeeding Education: Attend classes, workshops, informational sessions, support groups, and resources to enhance your knowledge, abilities, self-assurance, and readiness for breastfeeding. Gain insight into the physiology, positions, latch, feeding cues, difficulties, advantages, and practices that promote breastfeeding comfort, success, and well-being.

Consultation and Support: To address questions, concerns, plans, preparations, and individualized breastfeeding care to foster confidence, readiness, and empowerment for the breastfeeding journey, seek out prenatal lactation consultation, guidance, counseling, and support from lactation consultants, healthcare providers, counselors, educators, and breastfeeding advocates.

Breastfeeding a newborn and starting breastfeeding:

Immediate Skin-to-Skin Contact: Within the first hour following delivery, establish immediate skin-to-skin contact and breastfeeding to support early breastfeeding initiation, colostrum feeding, bonding, connection, warmth, comfort, and relaxation. These actions also help to promote breastfeeding success, initiation, and well-being in the mother-infant bonding and interaction domains.

Latch & Positioning: To help moms and babies have successful, comfortable, and successful breastfeeding experiences, milk transfer, and feeding sessions, practice and become an expert in breastfeeding positions, latches, holds, feeding signals, rhythms, patterns, and practices.

Feeding Cues and Responsive Feeding: Acknowledge and react to hunger cues, signs, and requirements of the newborn in order to start, continue, and end nursing sessions. This promotes responsive feeding, mother and baby comfort, and contentment throughout the day and night.

Help & Support for Breastfeeding:

Lactation Consultation and Guidance: Throughout the breastfeeding journey, transitions, and life stages, access lactation consultants, healthcare providers, support groups, counselors, educators, and breastfeeding advocates for ongoing lactation consultation, support, guidance, counseling, resources, and assistance with questions, concerns, adjustments, interventions, and support.

Peer Support and Community: Build relationships with other breastfeeding mothers, families, and advocates by getting involved in peer support groups, breastfeeding communities, forums, networks, and groups. By sharing experiences, insights, difficulties, triumphs, stories, resources, encouragement, and support, you can foster connection, empowerment, resilience, and well-being in the breastfeeding journey, community, and shared experiences.

Diet, hydration, and taking care of oneself:

Good Nutrition and Hydration: Throughout the breastfeeding journey and the postpartum period, maintain a balanced, nutrient-rich, and hydrating diet, lifestyle, and self-care practices to support optimal breastfeeding health, milk production, composition, supply, quality, maternal well-being, energy, vitality, recovery, and general health.

Rest, relaxation, and self-care: To support physical, emotional, psychological, and spiritual well-being, balance, resilience, recovery, energy, and positivity during breastfeeding, motherhood, and life transitions, embrace rest, relaxation, self-care, mindfulness, stress reduction, sleep, recuperation, and wellness practices.

The journey from conception to successful, comfortable, and fulfilling breastfeeding experiences, connections, interactions, and journeys between mothers and babies throughout infancy, growth, challenges, transitions, and life's unfolding chapters, all begin with embracing preparation, education, support, practice, connection, empowerment, resilience, patience, and holistic well-being. Encouraging safety, confidence, satisfaction, resilience, and well-being throughout the breastfeeding process, recovery, transformation, and life chapters can be achieved by actively participating in proactive, informed, personalized, attentive, and collaborative breastfeeding experiences, preparations, communications, consultations, evaluations, follow-ups, support, and care. It also celebrates connection, bonding, love, nurturing, empowerment, and the special journey of breastfeeding, motherhood, infancy, and life's evolving experiences. Accepting and valuing balance, comfort, connection, and the sacred journey of breastfeeding, motherhood, and life's unfolding adventures while embracing the breastfeeding journey with knowledge, readiness, support, empowerment, resilience, positivity, self-care, connection, and holistic well-being promotes healing, recovery, satisfaction, confidence, body positivity, life celebration, and thriving through individual and collective breastfeeding experiences, transformations, challenges, growth, and life chapters.

Typical Problems and Their Fixes

Even though it's healthy and natural, nursing can provide mothers and newborns with a number of hurdles as they go through the learning curve to create a successful breastfeeding practice. Mothers are more equipped to confront and overcome obstacles when they are aware of typical problems and possible solutions, which guarantees that nursing is enjoyable for both the mother and the child. Many breastfeeding difficulties can be successfully handled and resolved with time, encouragement, knowledge, and proactive problem-solving, promoting comfort, confidence, and overall wellbeing throughout the breastfeeding process.

CHAPTER THREE

Typical Breastfeeding Problems and Their Fixes:

Problems with Latch and Positioning:

Challenge: Inability to latch properly, resulting in pain, soreness, and discomfort in the nipples as well as inefficient milk transfer.

Solution: To ensure comfortable and successful nursing for mother and child, get advice from a lactation consultant or healthcare professional to evaluate and adjust latch techniques, positioning, holds, attachments, and feeding practices.

Low Supply of Milk:

Challenge: The frequency of feedings, milk production, satiety of the baby, and mother confidence are all impacted by the perceived or actual insufficient milk supply.

Solution: To maximize milk supply, breastfeeding success, and maternal well-being, increase the frequency of breastfeeding, make sure that milk removal is effective, practice skin-to-skin contact, use breast compression techniques, maintain hydration, nutrition, rest, and relaxation, and seek lactation consultation, support, guidance, and interventions.

Blocked Ducts and Engorgement:

Challenge: Blocked milk ducts, breast engorgement, fullness, swelling, pain, and tenderness that can lead to discomfort, make breastfeeding difficult, and increase the risk of infection.

Solution: To relieve engorgement, clear clogged ducts, and avoid mastitis, use frequent breastfeeding, efficient milk removal, warm compresses, light massage, breast compression, positioning adjustments, rest, hydration, pain management, and lactation consultation, support, guidance, and care.

Breast infections and mastitis:

Challenges include fever, flu-like symptoms, inflammation, redness, warmth, soreness, breast infections, and difficulties nursing.

Solution: To manage, treat, and prevent mastitis, infections, and complications, identify early symptoms, seek medical evaluation, diagnosis, treatment, antibiotics, rest, hydration, pain management, breastfeeding continuation, efficient milk removal, support, and guidance from healthcare providers, lactation consultants, and counselors.

Breast Pain and Injuries:

Challenge: Tenderness, discomfort, bleeding, blisters, trauma, pain in the breasts, cracks, and issues that make breastfeeding uncomfortable and enjoyable.

Solution: To promote healing, comfort, and happy breastfeeding experiences, address latch issues, positioning, attachment, breastfeeding techniques, pain management, nipple care, protection, healing, lanolin application, breast milk application, air drying, rest, support, guidance, and consultation from lactation specialists, healthcare providers, and counselors.

Feeding Difficulties and Infant Fears:

Challenges include: tongue-tie, lip-tie, jaundice, fussiness, latching troubles, weight issues, growth issues, and breastfeeding difficulties.

The best way to address and manage infant concerns, challenges, and feeding issues is to evaluate infant health, growth, feeding cues, weight gain, and feeding effectiveness. You can also seek medical evaluation, diagnosis, treatment, interventions, lactation consultation, support, guidance, feeding support, techniques, resources, and assistance from healthcare providers, pediatricians, lactation specialists, and counselors.

Overabundance of Milk and Quick Letdown:

Problème: An abundance of milk, rapid letdown response, vigorous milk flow, assuring the baby doesn't choke, gag, spit up, or get fussy as they feed.

Solution: To regulate milk supply, flow, and balance and optimize feeding comfort, effectiveness, and satisfaction for the mother and baby, manage breastfeeding positions, latch techniques, feeding cues, frequency, duration, block feeding, expressing milk, breast compression, reclined feeding positions, relaxation, support, guidance, consultation, and assistance from lactation consultants, healthcare providers, and counselors.

During the nursing journey, moms may face typical challenges related to breastfeeding. To effectively address, manage, and overcome these challenges, women need to receive understanding, support, education, proactive problem-solving, and collaborative care. Positive breastfeeding experiences, confidence, fulfillment, connection, bonding, and the nurturing journey of breastfeeding, motherhood, infancy, and life's unfolding adventures are fostered by embracing challenges with patience, resilience, empowerment, guidance, communication, assistance, and holistic well-being. In order to foster successful, comfortable, and fulfilling breastfeeding experiences, connections, interactions, and shared moments between mothers and babies throughout the breastfeeding journey, growth, transitions, and life's evolving chapters, it is important for women to seek timely, personalized, compassionate, and evidence-based care, support, resources, and interventions from healthcare providers, lactation consultants, counselors, and breastfeeding advocates. This celebrates the special, transformative, and sacred journey of breastfeeding, love, nurturing, resilience, and life's precious connections.

Diet and Nutrition for Nursing Mothers

In order to support breastfeeding moms' health, milk supply, composition, energy levels, recuperation, and general well-being throughout the postpartum phase, diet and nutrition are essential. Throughout the nursing journey, adopting a balanced, nutritious, and varied diet enhanced with vital nutrients, vitamins, minerals, hydration, and energy sources supports optimal health of the mother and her unborn child as well as the growth, development, and contentment of the mother.

Dietary Guidelines and Nutrition for Nursing Mothers:

Energy Needs and Caloric Intake:

Increased Calories: In order to maintain milk production, energy expenditure, metabolism, recuperation, and maternal wellbeing, breastfeeding moms need to consume extra calories. When breastfeeding, an additional 300–500 calories per day over pre-pregnancy intake is beneficial for milk synthesis, nutritional requirements, and energy demands.

Healthy Eating and Foods High in Nutrients:

Protein Sources: To support muscle repair, recuperation, milk production, and baby growth, include lean protein sources such as chicken, fish, eggs, dairy products, legumes, nuts, seeds, tofu, and plant-based proteins.

Healthy Fats: To support brain development, inflammation, immunity, hormone production, and milk composition, include omega-3 fatty acids, monounsaturated fats, polyunsaturated fats, and essential fatty acids found in fish, flaxseeds, chia seeds, walnuts, avocados, olive oil, nuts, and seeds.

Whole Grains and Carbohydrates: To provide sustained energy, fiber, vitamins, minerals, and nutrients for breastfeeding and maternal health, choose whole grains, complex carbohydrates, fruits, vegetables, and fiber-rich foods like oats, quinoa, brown rice, whole grain bread, pasta, cereals, and fruits and vegetables.

Calcium and Vitamin D: To support bone health, milk composition, and nutrient absorption during breastfeeding, eat foods high in calcium, such as dairy products, fortified plant-based milk, leafy greens, almonds, tofu, and salmon, along with foods high in vitamin D, such as supplements, fortified foods, and fatty fish.

Iron-Rich Foods: To support iron levels, energy, blood production, and lactation needs while nursing, include iron-rich foods such lean meats, chicken, fish, legumes, lentils, beans, tofu, spinach, and fortified cereals and grains.

Hydration: To boost milk production, hydration, metabolism, detoxification, and general health during breastfeeding, make sure you are getting enough water, herbal teas, decaffeinated beverages, and other fluids throughout the day.

Mineral and vitamin supplements:

Prenatal and Postnatal Supplements: Keep taking the prenatal vitamins, minerals, and supplements that your doctor has prescribed. These include calcium, vitamin D, iron, folic acid, and other vital nutrients that support milk production, breastfeeding, mother health, and the nutrition of the unborn child.

Avoiding Specific Foods and Drinks:

Limit Alcohol and Caffeine: To reduce exposure to, and potential effects on, the production of breast milk, the health of the infant, and the well-being of the mother while nursing, limit alcohol, stimulants, and caffeine intake. Instead, choose decaffeinated choices and practice moderation and safe consumption habits.

Allergens and Sensitivities: Keep an eye out for any possible allergies, sensitivities, reactions, or intolerances in the baby, including those to dairy, soy, nuts, gluten, and other foods. You can also monitor your child's diet and eliminate triggers by making dietary adjustments and seeking medical attention. Dietitians, lactation consultants, and healthcare professionals can also offer support and advice on breastfeeding issues, nutritional needs, and medical evaluations.

Meal Planning, Making, and Eating Snacks:

Meal Planning and Preparation: To support breastfeeding, appetite, cravings, and dietary preferences during the postpartum period, plan balanced meals, snacks, and nutrient-dense food options that are simple to prepare, convenient, accessible, and enjoyable. Incorporate variety, creativity, and flexibility in meal planning, recipes, and dietary practices.

Healthy Snacking: To sustain energy levels, satiate hunger, stabilize blood sugar, and support nursing demands throughout the day, embrace healthy snacking options like fruits, vegetables, nuts, seeds, yogurt, cheese, whole grains, smoothies, protein bars, and wholesome snacks.

The success of nursing, the health of the mother, the sustenance of the newborn, and the general well-being of the postpartum period all depend on diet and nutrition. Throughout the breastfeeding journey, transitions, and changing chapters of life, adopting a balanced, varied, nutrient-rich, and customized diet that incorporates vital nutrients, vitamins, minerals, hydration, and energy sources supports optimal breastfeeding health, milk production, composition, recovery, metabolism, energy levels, and satisfaction for mothers and babies. The nurturing journey of breastfeeding, motherhood, infancy, and life's precious moments are celebrated, along with the special, transformative, and sacred experiences of nourishment, love, growth, and connection throughout the breastfeeding journey and beyond. These outcomes are fostered by placing a high priority on self-care, mindfulness, nourishment, hydration, meal planning, preparation, support, consultation, and holistic well-being.

How to Pump and Store Breast Milk

For nursing moms who want to manage engorgement, share feeding duties with others, develop a milk supply, or provide breast milk while absent from their child, pumping and storing breast milk can be a helpful practice. The safety, quality, freshness, and nutritional integrity of expressed breast milk are ensured by appropriate pumping techniques, storage guidelines, handling procedures, and hygiene measures. These factors support the best possible milk supply, feeding, health, and well-being for moms and babies throughout the breastfeeding journey.

Breast milk pumping:

How to Choose a Breast Pump:

Manual or Electric Breast Pumps: Select a breast pump type according to your needs, preferences, comfort level, convenience of use, portability, flexibility in expressing breast milk, and frequency of pumping.

Pump Features: To choose a suitable pump that satisfies individual needs and supports efficient, comfortable, and convenient pumping experiences, take into account the pump's features, settings, speed, suction levels, flange sizes, comfort, noise level, portability, battery options, accessories, warranty, and reviews.

Pumping Methods & Approaches:

Clean Hands and Equipment: To maintain hygiene, safety, and milk quality, wash your hands thoroughly with soap and water. You should also make sure that the breast pump's parts, bottles, storage containers, and accessories are clean, sanitized, correctly constructed, and in good functioning order before pumping.

Comfortable Setting: To encourage milk flow, the let-down reflex, and comfort during pumping, create a calm, peaceful, quiet, and distraction-free environment for your sessions.

CHAPTER FOUR

You can do this by incorporating breathing exercises, music, visualization, mindfulness, relaxation techniques, and positive affirmations.

Pumping Schedule: To maximize milk production, storage, and utilization throughout the day and night, establish a consistent pumping schedule, frequency, duration, and timing that aligns with breastfeeding, infant feeding patterns, maternal routines, preferences, needs, milk supply goals, and breastfeeding support.

Breast Massage and Compression: To promote milk removal, stimulate milk flow, increase milk production, and provide comfort during breast milk expression, incorporate mild breast massage, compression, warm compresses, visualization, relaxation, and breast softening treatments before and during pumping sessions.

Keeping Explicit Breast Milk Stored:

Labels and Storage Containers:

Safe Containers: To preserve freshness, organization, and batch monitoring of milk, use clean, sanitized, BPA-free, food-grade bottles, storage bags, or freezer-safe containers made for storing and labeling expressed milk with date, time, and volume.

Storage Best Practices and Guidelines:

Room Temperature: If properly ventilated, shaded from the sun, and placed in a clean, covered container, newly expressed breast milk can be stored at room temperature (up to 77°F or 25°C) for up to 4-6 hours.

Refrigeration: To maintain freshness, quality, and nutritional content, refrigerate breast milk for up to 4–8 days at temperatures between 32°F and 39°F (0°C and 4°C) in the refrigerator's back, away from the door.

Freezing: To prevent contamination, freezer burn, odors, and temperature swings, store expressed breast milk in the freezer compartment (0°F or -18°C) for up to 6–12 months in a deep freezer or 3–6 months in a standard freezer. Use airtight, leak-proof, and freezer-safe storage bags, containers, or trays.

Warming and Thawing: To ensure safety, freshness, and comfort for the infant, gently thaw frozen breast milk in the refrigerator overnight or under cool running water. Before feeding, warm refrigerated or thawed milk to body temperature in a warm water bath (do not microwave); swirl gently.

Managing and Keeping Clean:

Clean Handling: To avoid contamination, spoilage, bacterial development, and health hazards for moms and babies, handle breast milk, containers, equipment, and accessories in a clean, sanitary, and safe manner during the pumping, storing, transporting, thawing, warming, and feeding procedures.

Labeling and Organization: Throughout breastfeeding, milk supply building, storage, and feeding practices, label, organize, rotate, and use breast milk batches based on storage dates to ensure first in, first out (FIFO) inventory management, freshness, quality, and optimal utilization of expressed milk.

Breastfeeding moms may manage engorgement, increase their milk supply, share feeding duties with others, and give breast milk when they are away from their babies with the flexibility and convenience that pumping and storing breast milk offers. The quality, freshness, nutrition, and integrity of expressed breast milk are ensured by adhering to recommended pumping techniques, storage guidelines, handling procedures, hygiene precautions, and safety measures. This promotes optimal breastfeeding experiences, milk production, supply, utilization, health, and well-being for mothers and babies throughout the breastfeeding journey, transitions, and life's evolving chapters. In order to foster successful, comfortable, and fulfilling breastfeeding practices, connections, bonding, and the nurturing journey of breastfeeding, motherhood, infancy, and life's precious moments, it is important to prioritize education, preparation, support, resources, consultation, collaboration, communication, self-care, and holistic well-being. This way, we can celebrate the special, transformative, and sacred experiences of breastfeeding, love, growth, and connection throughout the breastfeeding journey and beyond.

Nursing in Particular Situations

Special situations offer special challenges and considerations when it comes to breastfeeding. To address each mother and baby's unique needs, circumstances, medical conditions, and preferences throughout the breastfeeding journey, collaborative care, understanding, support, education, preparation, flexibility, and adaptability are essential. Fostering good experiences, empowerment, well-being, connection, bonding, and the nurturing journey of breastfeeding, maternity, infancy, and life's unfolding chapters is made possible by embracing individualized, compassionate, evidence-based, and holistic approaches to breastfeeding in exceptional situations.

Breastfeeding in Particular Situations:

Low birth weight or preterm babies:

NICU Support: Assist preterm or low birth weight infants with breastfeeding, kangaroo care, skin-to-skin contact, and lactation support by working together with neonatal intensive care unit (NICU) teams, lactation consultants, healthcare providers, nurses, and specialists. This involves attending to each baby's unique needs, feeding cues, challenges, health issues, and growth requirements.

Prioritize exclusive breastfeeding: For preterm or low birth weight infants, give special consideration to exclusive breast milk feeding, expressing breast milk, fortifying breast milk, tube feeding, syringe feeding, cup feeding, or bottle feeding as advised by health professionals, nutritional support, growth monitoring, and developmental milestones.

Medical Conditions and Medication Used by Mothers:

Consultation and Guidance: To address maternal medical conditions, medications, treatments, side effects, contraindications, and implications for breastfeeding, infant health, safety, nutrition, and well-being, seek individualised consultation, guidance, and collaboration with healthcare providers, specialists, lactation consultants, pharmacists, and counselors.

Medication Safety: To ensure safe, effective, and compatible breastfeeding practices, management, and care for mothers and babies with medical conditions, treatments, and medications, consider medication safety, risks, benefits, alternatives, timing, dosage, compatibility, monitoring, adjustments, and maternal-infant interactions.

Surrogacy, Adoption, or Induced Lactation:

Breastfeeding Support: To initiate, establish, and maintain breastfeeding or milk production for adopted or surrogate babies, explore options, techniques, protocols, hormone therapy, adoptive breastfeeding, induced lactation, relactation, and pumping. You can also get support from lactation consultants, healthcare providers, counselors, and specialists.

Nutritional Support: To improve milk production, quality, supply, bonding, and the nursing experience in adoption, surrogacy, or induced lactation journeys, prioritize proper nutrition, hydration, supplements, hormone treatment, galactagogues, support, education, and individualized care.

Breast Surgery, Anatomical Issues, or Difficulties with Breastfeeding:

Lactation Consultation: For advice on breast surgery, anatomical concerns, breastfeeding difficulties, latch issues, milk supply, infant feeding, and individualized breastfeeding strategies, solutions, and support, consult lactation consultants, healthcare professionals, surgeons, specialists, counselors, and support groups.

Alternative Feeding Techniques: To help with breastfeeding, milk transfer, comfort, and success in unique situations, investigate alternative feeding techniques, supplemental nursing systems (SNS), nipple shields, breast pumps, positioning, latch techniques, support aids, and resources.

Baby Health Issues, Allergies, or Particular Requirements:

Healthcare Collaboration: To address infant health concerns, allergies, special needs, feeding difficulties, nutritional requirements, formulas, dietary adjustments, and individualized breastfeeding or feeding strategies, support, and care, collaborate with pediatricians, specialists, allergists, dietitians, lactation consultants, and support groups.

Nutritional Management: In order to address infant health, growth, development, allergies, sensitivities, intolerances, and breastfeeding or feeding needs in unique situations, situations, and care settings, implement nutritional management, monitoring, evaluation, interventions, treatments, adjustments, and support.

Throughout the nursing journey, moms and babies have unique requirements, problems, situations, medical conditions, therapies, and preferences that must be addressed through individualized, compassionate, collaborative, knowledgeable, and adaptable approaches to breastfeeding in special circumstances. Nurturing positive breastfeeding experiences, connections, bonding, resilience, satisfaction, and the nurturing journey of breastfeeding, motherhood, infancy, and life's unfolding adventures in special circumstances, transitions, and chapters requires embracing supportive, flexible, evidence-based, holistic, and individualized care, communication, consultation, education, preparation, resources, empowerment, and well-being. Emphasizing knowledge, assistance, direction, advocacy, teamwork, self-care, self-compassion, patience, perseverance, and holistic well-being honors the many, transformative, and sacred breastfeeding experiences as well as love, connection, growth, and life's priceless moments during the breastfeeding journey as well as unique situations, difficulties, joys, and beyond.

Weaning and Leaving Breastfeeding Behind

A major milestone, weaning and quitting breastfeeding require careful planning, gradual adjustments, emotional support, communication, understanding, patience, flexibility, and respect for the readiness, needs, preferences, and developmental stages of the mother and child throughout the process. Supporting positive experiences, comfort, bonding, emotional well-being, and the nurturing journey of switching from breastfeeding to alternative feeding methods, as well as independence and new chapters in the mother-child relationship and family dynamics, are all facilitated by embracing compassionate, responsive, and personalized approaches to weaning.

Transitioning from Breastfeeding to Weaning:

Evaluating Preferences and Readiness:

Mother and Child Readiness: Determine whether the mother and child are physically, emotionally, socially, and developmentally ready for weaning. Pay attention to cues, signals, changes, interests, behaviors, and preferences that show comfort, openness, and readiness for weaning, transition, and feeding pattern changes.

Gradual and Gentle Approach: Throughout the weaning process, take a gradual, gentle, and patient approach, respecting the individual preferences, pacing, comfort levels, and responses of both mother and child. This will foster collaboration, understanding, communication, connection, bonding, and trust.

Techniques and Strategies for Weaning:

Reduce nursing: Gradually reduce, space out, or decrease nursing sessions, feedings, times, lengths, and frequency over time to provide comfort, adjustment, and adaption while switching from breastfeeding to other feeding practices, routines, and methods.

Substitution and Alternatives: To replace nursing, introduce alternate feeding techniques, routines, bottles, cups, solids, and milk sources. Give them choices, variety, and autonomy when it comes to feeding, caring, bonding, and trying out new weaning and transition experiences.

Comfort, Support, and Diversion: During the weaning process, offer comfort, emotional support, reassurance, distraction, activities, bonding, closeness, and connection. Address emotions, feelings, changes, and transitions with comprehension, empathy, patience, creativity, and positive reinforcement.

Psychological and Emotional Assistance:

In order to promote security, trust, comfort, and positive experiences in the mother-child relationship, bonding, and transitions, it is important to cultivate emotional bonding, connection, closeness, cuddling, skin-to-skin contact, quality time, reassurance, presence, responsiveness, and affection during the weaning process.

Communication and Understanding: Throughout the weaning process, acknowledge, validate, and respect the child's viewpoints, reactions, curiosity, and responses. Talk about weaning, changes, feelings, emotions, expectations, boundaries, alternatives, and transitions in an open, sensitive, age-appropriate, and honest manner.

Sustaining Physical and Nutritional Health:

Nutritional Transition: To satisfy nutritional needs, growth, development, health, and well-being during and after weaning from breastfeeding, ensure a smooth nutritional transition, balance, diversity, adequacy, and intake of age-appropriate meals, beverages, supplements, and feeding habits.

Physical Comfort and Well-Being: Throughout the weaning process, provide comfort measures, pain relief, care, guidance, and individualized attention to support physical well-being, health, recovery, and comfort. Attend to physical comfort, adjustments, responses, reactions, changes, needs, and support.

Honoring and Celebrating the Weaning Process:

Positivity in Reflection and Celebration: Throughout the breastfeeding and weaning chapters, transitions, and life's unfolding adventures, celebrate, honor, acknowledge, and cherish the weaning journey, milestones, accomplishments, growth, changes, connections, bonding, shared moments, experiences, and memories.

The process of weaning and quitting breastfeeding is complex and requires a variety of skills, including patience, flexibility, empathy, creativity, and respect for the needs, preferences, readiness, and developmental stages of the mother and child at each stage of the process. In the mother-child relationship, family dynamics, and shared experiences throughout the weaning journey, transitions, and beyond, adopting compassionate, responsive, personalized, and nurturing approaches to weaning fosters positive experiences, comfort, bonding, emotional well-being, resilience, trust, connection, and the transformative journey of moving from breastfeeding to alternative feeding methods, independence, new beginnings, and life's evolving chapters. The weaning process, connections, memories, growth, love, and the priceless moments of breastfeeding, motherhood, infancy, childhood, and life's unfolding adventures are nurtured by placing a high priority on understanding, support, patience, empowerment, self-care, reflection, celebration, and holistic well-being. Transitions, challenges, joys, and milestones are celebrated in the heartwarming journey of love, connection, and the beautiful evolution of motherhood and child development.

Summary

In summary, nursing is a special and private experience that has many advantages for moms and infants. It strengthens a unique link, gives vital nutrients, boosts the growth of the immune system, and provides security and comfort. Moms can better handle the joys and challenges of nursing when they are aware of the anatomy, physiology, and dynamics of the process.

It's important to keep informed about breast health, from knowing the architecture and physiology of the breast to knowing the various types of breast cancer and disorders. Effective management of breast problems, improvement of prognosis, and promotion of well-being are contingent upon early identification, diagnosis, and treatment.

In order to preserve their health and promote milk supply, breastfeeding moms should place a high priority on diet, water, and self-care. When breast milk is pumped and stored properly, newborns can continue to receive healthy meals even when they are taken away from their moms.

Personalized approaches to breastfeeding are necessary in special circumstances, such as preterm birth, medical issues, or a history of surgery, to ensure the safety, comfort, and best health of both mother and child. The important milestone of weaning from breastfeeding should be handled sensitively, gradually, and with understanding, taking into account the individual needs and preparedness of both mother and child.

Consulting with healthcare professionals, lactation consultants, counselors, and support groups can be a great way to get advice, comfort, and encouragement along the way. In addition to celebrating the life-changing experience of motherhood, growth, connection, and the shared moments of love, care, and nurturing throughout life's beautiful chapters and milestones, embracing the difficulties and joys of breastfeeding with patience, resilience, compassion, and love strengthens the bond between mother and child.

THE END